Table of Contents

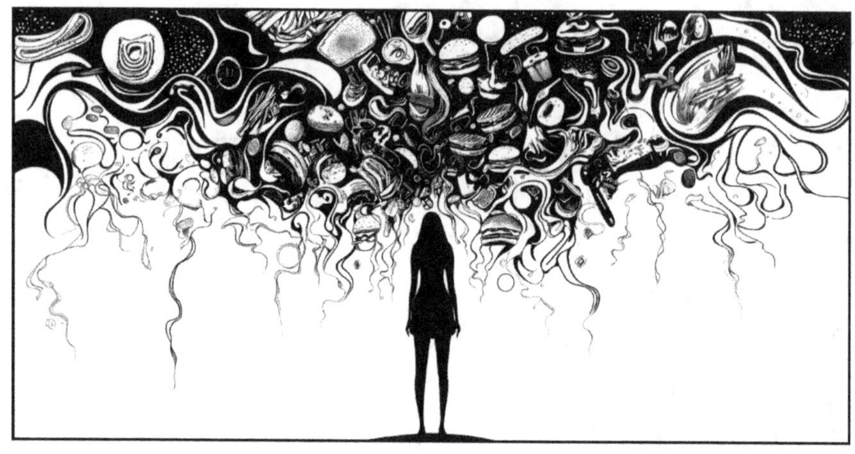

Introduction — «Welcome to My Calorie Nightmare»

My name is Hannah, I'm 36 years old, and I've decided to write this book for those who feel a bit lost in this life. There was a time when I was on the brink of despair. I want you to know: you are not alone in your struggles. There are times when it feels like everything is going wrong, and each new day is just a replay of yesterday's nightmare. But believe me, any problem can be overcome.

When I look at my reflection in the mirror, I see not only my current body but the entire journey that brought me here—a journey from 247 pounds to 123 pounds. It was a long and difficult path, full of disappointments, pain, and doubts. But at the same time, it was a journey to myself, to the realization that I deserved better. I went through a lot: from dull days in the office to personal crises and turmoil, where each new day felt like an extension of yesterday's nightmare. But the main thing I realized is this: even when it seems like there's no way out, there's always a chance to come to a new version of yourself—stronger and more confident.

In this book, I will share my story—not perfect, but real, full of mistakes and unexpected twists. A story of how I went from indifference and despair to realizing that I needed to take control of my life and start making changes. You'll see that if I could overcome my demons, so can you. Yes, it won't be easy. There are moments when you just want to quit and give up, but it's precisely in those moments that you need to find the strength to keep going.

My life was like most people's: work, home, occasional weekends. Each new day resembled the previous one, and this endless routine gradually pushed everything else out. In the morning, I would wake up, get ready for work, and already knew what lay ahead—the same tasks, the same faces, and it all seemed to repeat in a loop. In the office, my duties had long ceased to be interesting. Routine tasks filled my entire day—working with databases, checking ads, cleaning up duplicates. But in some way, it became familiar, even comforting. It was my microcosm, where everything moved at its own pace.

However, despite the boredom of the work itself, the team was what added some positive notes to this monotony. We could laugh at the ridiculous mistakes in the ads or discuss the latest news. Simple conversations with colleagues, jokes, and discussions helped distract from monotonous assignments and liven up the day a bit. Each of us played our part in this work «theater,» and the team really made life brighter, if only for a short while.

But when the workday ended, I found myself back in the routine. Evenings at home with my boyfriend became just as predictable as the weekdays at the office. We talked about the same things—household chores, shopping lists, plans for the next day. Everything boiled down to monotony, and it seemed like nothing was changing. Our rare outings to cafes or bars with his friends were perhaps the only chance to get out of the house. But even those moments didn't bring joy. I would listen to the conversations but didn't feel like I was part of them. Everything revolved around his friends, their jokes, and memories in which I had no place. And although I was in the company of others, I still felt lonely.

Sometimes it felt like my life was moving in a closed loop, with no way out in sight. The office routine and the monotony of personal life overlapped, amplifying the feeling of helplessness. Any attempts to change something yielded no results—neither at work nor at home. The only bright spot that gave me a fleeting sense of joy was food. Delicious food became a small consolation, a source of pleasure in this endless grayness. Life around me continued to move forward, but I seemed stuck, watching from the sidelines as everything moved on but didn't change. At that time, I didn't know that a serious challenge was awaiting me, one that would make me reconsider everything that had come before.

That was my starting point to 247 pounds, and then back to 123 pounds. I went through moments of despair when it felt like every step forward changed nothing. But at some point, something inside me changed. I decided to fight, no matter how hard it was. This journey was my personal challenge, and now, looking back, I realize that it wasn't just about the weight—it was about reclaiming control over my life. This book is not just a story about battling extra pounds; it's a story about how I found myself again. I managed to do it, and so can you. The main thing is not to be afraid to take the first step, no matter how small it may be.

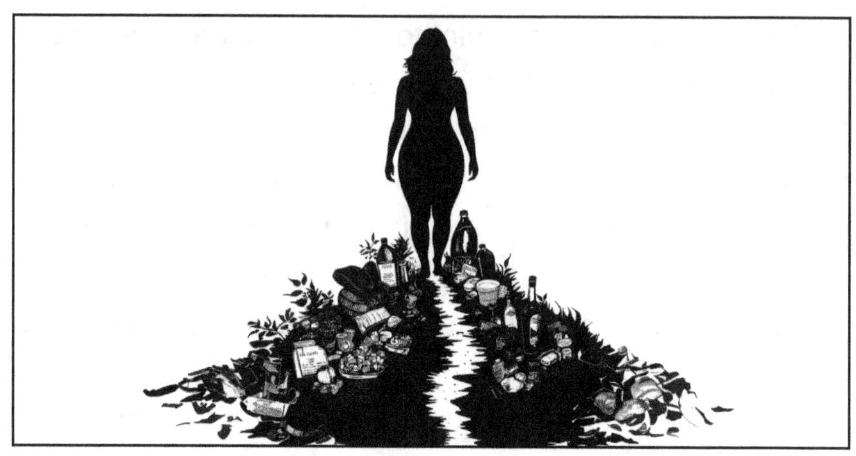

Chapter 1 — «How I Let This Weight Chaos Begin»

Late dinners became a ritual for us. When he came home late, I was already preparing dinner, which I thought was the perfect way to end our day. But who could have thought that these cozy evenings with a fragrant dish on the table and our favorite TV show on the screen would be the beginning of my journey to the 247-pound mark. It wasn't just about the food; it was the time we spent together, a way to escape and drown out the worries of the day. In those moments, I felt like I was in control of my life, providing comfort for both of us. Alcohol also became an integral part of our dinners. Beer with nuts and chips became our signature dish, symbolizing our time together. Sometimes it seemed that the crunch of the nuts was the only real sound in our quiet home, dispelling the silence and creating an illusion of closeness.

My mom, of course, noticed the changes happening to me. «Hannah, you've gained weight,» she would say with a touch of sadness in her voice. I saw the look in her eyes, full of care and concern, but I brushed it off every time: «Mom, it's all under control.» I tried to believe those words myself. But in reality, nothing was under control. My boyfriend noticed that I had gained weight too, but he kept silent, though his eyes said it all. Every time I tried to fit into my favorite jeans, I saw his barely noticeable disappointment. Clothes were becoming looser, not because I was losing weight, but because I was buying things in bigger sizes. And then the day came when I reached the largest size in the store. A wave of shame washed over me, and I realized that this couldn't go on any longer.

I decided that something needed to change, but where to start? The gym seemed like the logical solution. It's the place where people change their lives, and I decided I could too. I bought a membership and started going. The first few months were filled with enthusiasm and determination. Each workout was like a battle with my inner demons. The result? There was some, but not the one I hoped for. I lost some weight, but nothing significant. However, I began to feel physically stronger. I enjoyed the feeling of exhaustion after a workout when my muscles ached as if proving that I was really doing something. Every time the trainer talked about nutrition, I nodded, pretending to agree, but inside I laughed: «How can you give up your favorite food? It's a part of me!»

At the same time, I tried cooking separately for myself. A

salad for me, grilled chicken for him. But every time I smelled the freshly cooked chicken, my intentions crumbled. In the end, I made two portions: one for him and one for myself. And everything was eaten to the last crumb. I justified myself: «I'm eating salad, and the trainer allowed chicken!» But the truth was, the trainer meant a different kind of chicken, not the one I roasted with butter and spices, creating a crispy crust.

The crisis in the relationship with my boyfriend only worsened the situation. We argued more and more, and instead of seeking support from him, I sought it in food. Food became my refuge, my way to escape problems and loneliness. Each of our quarrels ended with another trip to the refrigerator. He lay on the couch, lost in his thoughts, while I tried to find comfort in food. Sometimes it felt like the refrigerator was the only one always ready to accept me. At some point, I realized that I couldn't go on like this. We broke up.

The breakup opened up a lot of free time, which seemed to have nothing to fill. Instead of channeling that energy into something useful, I found solace in alcohol and endless gatherings with friends. Every evening turned into a mini-party. My friends were happy: «Finally, you're back with us! Let's drink to a new life!» We laughed, chatted, ordered pizza, and it became our new ritual. «Now you can do anything,» they said, and I believed them, allowing myself everything I wanted. This «new» lifestyle included unlimited calories.

None of us thought about proper nutrition or workouts. It was a time of freedom, and I, as if freed from chains, dove into it headfirst. Every day became a calorie nightmare. First one cocktail, then a second, and by midnight, the table was filled with empty bottles and plates. «Why deny yourself pleasure?» I convinced myself, sending another piece of chocolate cake into my mouth.

My figure continued to grow, and with it, my appetite increased. Instead of the gym, I chose cafes, bars, and restaurants. Convincing myself that I deserved rest and pleasure after all my suffering, I plunged even deeper into this whirlwind of food and drinks. «Life should be bright!» I repeated, taking another serving of fries, assuring myself that this was happiness. And so, several months passed.

However, gradually, I realized that despite the parties and the seeming freedom, my weight kept growing. The short episode with the gym now seemed like just an illusion, an attempt to deceive myself. I still wasn't ready to stop and rethink my lifestyle. I continued to seek solace in food and alcohol until one day, flipping through my old photos, I noticed that I once thought of myself as «full,» but now those pictures became an unattainable ideal of slimness.

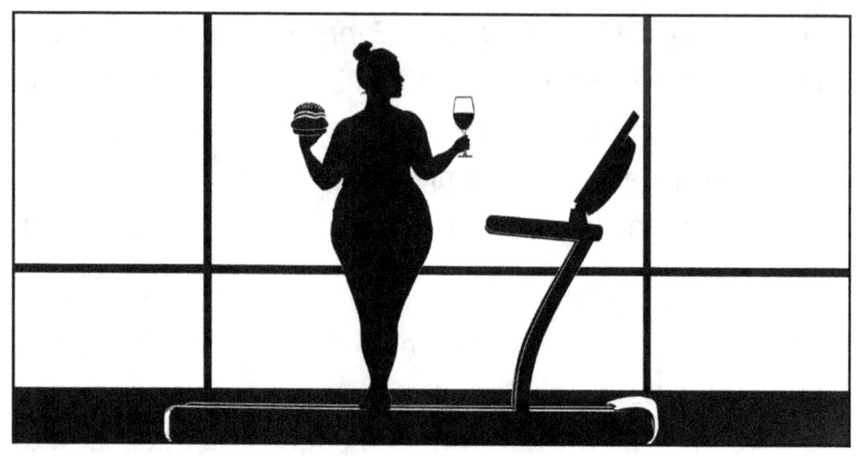

Chapter 2 — «My Body Against Me: The Battle Continues»

With new thoughts that now, without a partner, losing weight would be easier and that I only needed to cook for myself, I decided to continue my fight. It seemed like I would have more time for myself, to focus on my health. I imagined long walks, quiet evenings with a cup of herbal tea, and light salads, but reality turned out to be different. Soon, I faced an unexpected challenge—having more free time that was no longer filled with the usual interactions with my partner. This free time quickly became occupied by friends and frequent meetups, and along with them came the return of alcohol-fueled parties. At first, these were rare gatherings, but they soon turned into regular events that were hard to resist. Although there was less food at these meetups, alcohol, which is terribly high in calories, became the new problem. It often seemed like a couple of glasses of wine wouldn't hurt, but these gatherings eventually turned into real feasts. Pizza, chips, and other «party» foods became constant companions, and I found myself trapped again.

Moreover, the consequences of several years of overeating were starting to show. I realized that my stomach was stretched, and one apple was no longer enough to satisfy my hunger for even 20 minutes—I had to eat at least three or four. This realization didn't come to me immediately. For a long time, I wondered why the usual portions that should have satisfied me left me feeling unfulfilled. This discovery led to another round of self-analysis, but instead of addressing the issue, I delved further into a new lifestyle where alcohol and random snacks became the norm. Deep down, I knew something was wrong, but I was afraid to admit it to myself.

In 2011, I decided to make a drastic change in my career and quit my office job, hoping that working remotely for an international IT company would not only provide a stable income but also give me the chance to focus more on my health. It seemed that remote work was an excellent option: more free time, no need to spend hours commuting to the office. I dreamed that now I could visit the gym at convenient times, walk more in the fresh air, and cook healthy food. But in practice, it led to even less physical activity. I spent entire days sitting at the computer, only getting up to walk to the fridge. Each trip to the fridge felt like a mini-adventure, a distraction from the monotony of the day, and I began to notice that I was using food to fill the void that office work used to occupy.

Health problems began to accumulate. I increasingly felt weak, joint pain became constant, and headaches and fever were a regular occurrence. It was as if my body was sending me distress signals, which I ignored. Elevated blood sugar levels caused concern, and after consulting an endocrinologist, I was diagnosed with metabolic syndrome. This meant that my body was already struggling to cope with the stress, and serious treatment was necessary. The endocrinologist prescribed medication and recommended following a strict 1,500-calorie diet. My new diet allowed green vegetables, lean meat, eggs, and a limited amount of fruit, completely excluding sweets, alcohol, fried, and fatty foods. These restrictions initially seemed almost impossible, as they affected not just habits but my social life too. How could I socialize with friends without a glass of wine? How could I enjoy the weekends without my favorite «unhealthy» treats?

Despite all the recommendations, my life was full of temptations. Constant parties and alcohol consumption interfered with my ability to stick to the diet. There were days when I thought I could control everything, that one night out wouldn't hurt. But each time, it turned out to be just self-deception. Although I regularly went to the gym, trying to find a balance between my desires and the need to take care of my health, the situation did not improve. Every workout became a test of endurance, both physical and mental. I often thought, «Is it even worth continuing if it doesn't work out anyway?» However, I understood that physical activity was one of the few ways to improve my condition and help my body cope with the stress I was putting it through.

Medical recommendations were strict: I needed to follow not just the diet but also take the medication prescribed by the endocrinologist to control my blood sugar levels and improve my metabolism. The medication helped to some extent, reducing the most acute symptoms, but they didn't solve the problem. Blood pressure spikes, joint pain, and headaches became unbearable, and every day was a struggle with my own body. I realized that I needed to make a drastic lifestyle change but was afraid to admit that in this process, I was my own worst enemy.

Once again, I came to the realization that this couldn't go on. Every day seemed like an endless repetition of the same scenario: overeating, feeling guilty, and making empty promises to start over tomorrow. But tomorrow came, and nothing changed. It was as if all my attempts to change my life were hitting an invisible wall that I had built myself. I realized I was in a vicious cycle that I needed to break out of before it was too late. It was an endless struggle with myself, where each day ended in defeat and disappointment.

The next pair of jeans that wouldn't button up became my wake-up call. These weren't just jeans—they were a symbol of all my attempts and failures, my entire journey in the fight against weight. They hung in my closet as a reminder of what I needed to do for myself, of how I owed it to myself to get my health and body back. I went back to the endocrinologist I had already known, who strongly recommended not just watching my diet but also maintaining a regular level of physical activity. He explained that to improve my condition and lose weight, regular physical exercises and a strict diet were necessary. This time, his words sounded like an ultimatum. I realized I was on the brink, and this was my last chance to change the situation.

After another visit to the doctor, I got a call from my friends inviting me to go out. I felt that I needed support and social interaction, so I immediately agreed, hoping for a calm evening. I imagined evening talks in the fresh air, light jokes, and a relaxing atmosphere that would help distract me from all the problems. I wanted to believe that I could spend time with my friends without breaking my new rules. However, a small sense of unease settled inside me, a slight fear that everything would once again go according to the usual scenario.

And my anxiety was not unfounded. We ended up at our favorite bar, where the atmosphere quickly pulled me into its rhythm. As soon as we walked in, the tables started filling up with cocktails, beer, and snacks. Inside, I froze with the desire to join in the fun. It seemed like here, in this noisy and vibrant place, all problems could disappear, if only for a few hours. I tried to hold on, reminding myself of the doctor's recommendations and my own promises. But the temptation was stronger. As soon as I let go of control, the evening turned into a whirlwind of events: laughter, music, bright lights—all of it drawing me deeper and deeper into the atmosphere of uninhibited fun. And at that moment, I found myself taking a step back in my fight for a better future.

After every such evening, I would promise myself once again that this couldn't continue. But after my evening workout, I would call my friends again, asking where the next meetup would be. As soon as I walked out of the gym feeling a sense of accomplishment, within a couple of hours, I would find myself at a party, immersed in the same atmosphere I was so desperately trying to escape. This cycle became like a closed loop, from which it seemed there was no way out. I realized that there was no progress towards the better, but I was comforted by the fact that at least I wasn't gaining any more weight.

Indeed, my weight remained stable, and this gave me a false sense of stability. It seemed like I wasn't losing weight, but I wasn't gaining either, and this became a kind of consolation for me. I started convincing myself that adapting to a new lifestyle would take time and that soon I would see real changes. The doctor's words, countless articles, and advice from the internet all talked about the need for patience, and I clung to this idea like a lifeline. But despite all the promises to myself, I continued to break the routine and found myself in the same situation, justifying it by saying, «everything is under control.»

I kept convincing myself that changes take time and that every small step forward was already a victory. I told myself that getting used to a new lifestyle couldn't be quick, and I needed to be patient. But the longer I went down this path, the clearer it became: I was stuck in the same trap of self-deception. Instead of fighting for a better future, I unconsciously continued on the familiar path, justifying every step back. I still hoped for the best, but the fear of real change kept me in this cycle. I was afraid that if I took a real step forward, I would have to face the things I had been avoiding for so long: real problems, real pain, and, most importantly, myself.

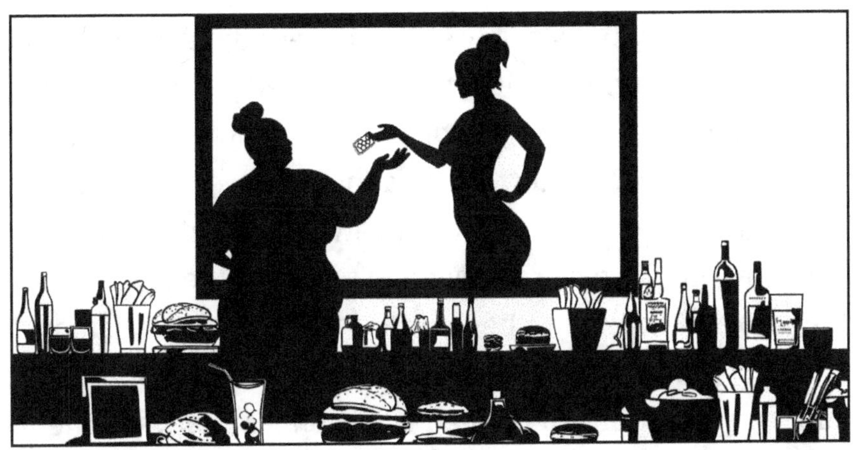

Chapter 3 — «Diets? Isn't that just another form of torture?»

I started looking back more and more, reflecting on all my attempts and failures. Each memory brought a sense of shame and disappointment, like a heavy stone pulling me down. At first, I believed that diets and exercise would truly help. I was full of enthusiasm: I studied the caloric content of foods, developed detailed workout plans, and eagerly stocked up on «right» foods. I was sure that this time it would work. But each time, my plans fell apart like a house of cards in a gust of wind. I tried to understand where I went wrong, looking for excuses, convincing myself that I just hadn't found «my» way. However, the longer I tried, the clearer it became—it wasn't about the method, it was about me.

New attempts were replaced by old mistakes. I began experimenting with diets, testing my endurance, as if I was testing my body's limits. There were days when I only drank water, and other days when I lived on yogurt, as if that could bring the long-awaited result. Sometimes, I went to extremes, completely eliminating carbs or fats, hoping that such a sacrifice would be rewarded. But the more I experimented, the worse my condition became. Weakness, fatigue, and irritability became my constant companions. My body could no longer cope, and my mind refused to accept new attempts; it seemed to no longer believe in them. But I continued, as if expecting that these difficulties were temporary and the result would come soon. It was like I was backing myself into a corner, hoping for a miracle.

Each failure gradually took away my hope. With each new failure, it became harder to believe that I would ever achieve my goal. I saw no point in these attempts but couldn't stop. There was still a spark inside me, reaching for the idea that I could change if I didn't give up. It became an addiction—I knew I was hurting myself, but I kept going. It seemed to me that if I stopped now, it would be the final defeat, and I couldn't allow myself to lose after all the years and effort spent.

Gradually, I began to realize that my struggle wasn't so much with my weight as it was with myself. Each new diet, each workout wasn't an attempt to change my body but to prove to myself that I could be better, stronger, more disciplined. It was a battle with my own demons, with fears and insecurities that held me back. But each time, I remained the same—with those fears and insecurities. It was as if I was fighting my own reflection, and every time I lost. My body became my enemy, and I didn't know how to come to terms with it, how to accept it.

This despair started to make me angry at myself. I had allowed my weight to become the center of my life. How many times had I given up simple joys for the sake of diets and workouts? How many times had I canceled meetings with friends, avoided family celebrations because there was food and I was afraid of breaking down? And all for what? Every step I took seemed wrong, every mistake—fatal. I was angry at myself for my weakness, for choosing the easy path, and allowing myself to compromise. But the more angry I became, the deeper I sank into this endless feeling of guilt.

There came a moment when I realized I could no longer continue this path. One day, I looked in the mirror and saw a completely unfamiliar person. I no longer recognized myself. In my eyes, I saw pain and disappointment. Every attempt seemed pointless, and the thought of a new diet or workout was revolting. I was exhausted to the limit, both physically and mentally. It was as if all my strength had been drained, and there was nothing left to keep me going.

Once again, desperate and realizing that endless workouts at the gym weren't yielding the desired results, I began to think about how to defeat this insatiable appetite that made me eat everything in sight. Every day turned into a struggle: workouts, attempts to stick to a diet plan, and then the inevitable breakdown when I would greedily pounce on food. It seemed that all my efforts were in vain. In search of answers,

I turned to the internet, where you can find everything at once—from diet plans to miraculous ways to curb appetite.

Hundreds of articles, thousands of tips, countless comments from people who had gone through the same thing. It seemed everyone knew the best way to deal with the problem, but in reality, it all came down to the same advice: «Control yourself,» «Stick to the plan,» «Don't overeat.» But what if you're hungry? Really hungry... How can you control this feeling when it becomes overwhelming? These questions seemed to go unanswered. The more I tried to restrain myself, the stronger my appetite became. And as if hearing my pleas, the internet started bombarding me with ads for miraculous pills. These pills promised everything: from appetite suppression to instant weight loss. «Buy this—go to sleep and wake up as a slender beauty,» they promised.

This advertising haunted me everywhere: on social media, news sites, even in my email newsletters. I knew such miraculous remedies were a scam, that you can't just lose weight by taking a pill. But the longer I weighed the pros and cons, the more I began to doubt. What if it really works? I tried to fight my appetite as doctors recommended: drink more water, eat small portions, avoid stress. But none of this worked. It seemed that every meal turned into a new battle, and in the end, I would lose. Months passed, and the weight stayed the same. Inside me, the frustration grew. I looked in the mirror and saw no changes. Another attempt had failed, leaving a bitter taste in my soul. It seemed that even trying to lead a healthy lifestyle wasn't yielding results.

At one point, I snapped. I saw yet another ad for a miracle cure and, unable to hold back, decided to order it. «Why not give it a try?» I thought. The bottle of miracle pills arrived a few days later. I started taking them as directed. Day after day, I took these pills, hoping for a miracle. A month passed, but there was no result. Neither did my appetite diminish, nor did the weight go away. Every day, I woke up expecting that everything would change, but in the mirror, I saw the same picture. Nothing had changed: my appetite remained, and so did my weight. The only thing I could be glad about was that at least there was no harm. But instead of joy, I accumulated even more disappointment, and each day this inner emptiness became more tangible. With this feeling, the pills were thrown into the trash. «You knew it wouldn't work, so what were you hoping for?» I thought. This thought left an unpleasant aftertaste. I knew it wouldn't work, but I still bought it, still tried.

Several more years passed, and I stumbled upon another remedy that promised even greater miracles. I read many reviews and articles about this drug. Analyzing its mechanism of action, I concluded that it should work. Unlike the previous pills, this one seemed more scientific and fact-based. It wasn't just promises—it seemed like something more serious. I was sure I had found what I was looking for. But the more I delved into the information, the more one word began to worry me: «poison.» This remedy was extremely dangerous. It was a real toxin, and its misuse could lead to horrible consequences. There was even a detailed guide online on how to take it to lose weight without getting poisoned. At first, I was shocked, but despite this, I decided to take the risk.

After three days of taking the pills, I began to notice the first effects: my appetite really decreased. But along with this came strange side effects. I constantly felt hot, as if I had a fever. My body was covered in sticky sweat with an unpleasant yellowish tint, and weakness literally enveloped me. Every step was a huge effort, but I continued to hope for a miracle. Inside, I convinced myself: «You have to endure; the result is near.» But after a few more days, my condition worsened: red spots began to appear on my skin, especially on my joints, and one of my friends noticed that my eyes had turned yellow. He looked at me with concern and said, «Hannah, stop this immediately! It's dangerous!» Inside, everything sank. His words sounded like a cold shower. I realized it was time to stop. My expectations were shattered, and disappointment filled the void I had been trying to fill with these attempts.

I stopped taking the remedy, but the recovery process was slow. The feeling of heat and weakness didn't go away for several days, and I felt completely drained. My body was recovering, and along with it, my thoughts were coming back to life. At that moment, I began to think about what I was doing with my life. Each failed attempt to lose weight left me with less and less hope. It was like an endless battle in which I always lost. And although I was no longer taking dangerous pills, I still couldn't get rid of the guilt. I was haunted by the disappointment: how could I take such a risk for a dubious result? I knew it could be dangerous, but I still took that step.

Every time I looked at my reflection in the mirror, waves of self-criticism engulfed me. How could I reach a point where even poisons seemed like acceptable means to achieve my goal? The internal dialogue didn't stop for a minute: «How could you be so foolish?» «Were you really ready to go that far?» These questions gave me no peace. I tried to convince myself that I was just desperate, that I was trying to do everything I could, but it didn't help. My head was full of so many questions, but not one answer could bring any comfort.

I tried to return to normal life again, but every time I tried something new to lose weight, I was haunted by a sense of doom. It seemed that every step I took led only to more failure. I felt trapped, with no way out. Everything I did seemed meaningless. Every new diet, every new attempt to control my appetite—all of it was useless. Everything fell apart, leaving a feeling of deep inner emptiness.

In moments of such reflection, I was overwhelmed by a sense of emptiness. Inside, there was no faith or hope left that I could change my life for the better. All my attempts to lose weight ended in disappointment, and I saw no point in continuing. I was spending more and more energy fighting with myself, and in the end—nothing. My body remained the same, and every day I felt that I was losing not only physical strength but also inner strength. I began to wonder why I was so persistently going down this path if I always ended up in the same place.

I began to question why I had tried all this time. All this struggle, all this effort, all these sacrifices—for what? I couldn't find an answer. It seemed to me that the world around me was moving forward, and I was staying in place. I felt like a failure. No diet, no exercise, no pill could change the fact that I remained the same. All my dreams of losing weight collapsed one by one like a house of cards. Each unsuccessful attempt left less and less hope.

This time, I couldn't even make myself smile or find any positive aspect in my situation. All I saw was an endless cycle of attempts and failures. I was sure I had exhausted all my resources, all my strength. Inside, there was emptiness, as if I had lost all my bearings. This time, I just sat down and allowed myself to cry. I realized that I had reached the point where I could no longer continue. All I had left was to admit my defeat and come to terms with the fact that perhaps losing weight wasn't my destiny.

Gradually, a thought began to form inside me that maybe I should stop fighting with myself and accept who I am. Acceptance didn't come immediately, but it slowly enveloped me like a warm blanket on a cold day. Yes, I didn't reach the ideal I had envisioned, but maybe that's okay? Maybe it's worth learning to live in harmony with myself rather than in constant struggle? Accepting my body seemed like a difficult task, but it became a new stage for me. Acceptance brought with it a quiet but tangible freedom from the pressure I had placed on myself.

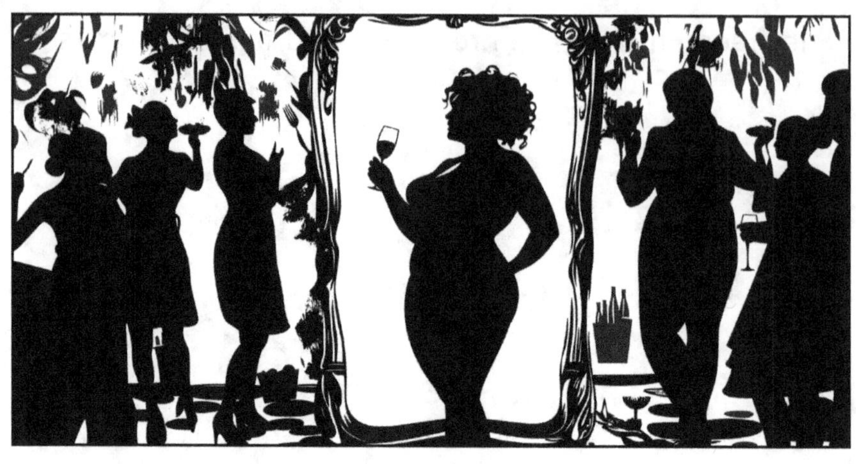

Chapter 4 — «Friends and Foes: Alcohol and Parties»

After long and often exhausting thoughts about my end-less failures with diets and pills, I realized it was time to radically change my approach to life. In previous years, I was constantly battling with myself, my weight, and a deep sense of guilt over my own shortcomings. Every new day felt like another test, where I tried again and again to fit into other people's standards, which seemed unreachable. Every diet, every new eating plan, or workout turned into an attempt to deceive myself, and each time I failed. But then came a moment of realization—I understood that this was a pointless and exhausting battle with windmills. I no longer aspired to be someone else, nor did I dream of waking up the next day slim and carefree. It felt like an acceptance of the inevitable—an understanding that I didn't have to meet others' expectations. Instead of wasting energy on fruitless attempts to change, I decided to channel it into something that could truly bring benefit. Thoughts about my weight still lingered somewhere in the depths of my mind, like an echo of the past, but they were no longer the main driving force of my life. From that moment on, I started to create my life according to my own script, not the one society imposed on me.

To distract myself from the oppressive feeling of failure in every aspect of my life, I decided to pour all my energy into work. I needed to prove to myself that I was capable of more than just losing endless battles with my body. Work became the very field where I could realize my ambitions and feel in control of my fate. I took on more responsibilities than before, and I noticed how my relationships with colleagues and bosses began to change. They started to trust me with more complex tasks, and with that came respect. Work became a source of stability, the very sense of security I lacked in my personal life. I could spend hours on projects, dissecting them down to the smallest details, and I didn't even stop working on weekends. Every completed task gave me a sense of victory that I had been deprived of for so long. I began to see that I could be successful in other areas, and this gave me confidence that my life was indeed moving forward.

My career became more than just a way to make money; it was a lifeline that made me feel like I wasn't lost in life. Colleagues began to respect me for my professionalism and diligence, and my bosses for my responsibility and dedication. It was exactly what I needed. I worked late, sometimes even into the night, burying myself in tasks to keep the thoughts of my internal failures from creeping back in. Work became my refuge, a place where I could prove to myself and others that I was capable of more. My career successes became a beacon, lighting the path I could lean on when everything else seemed too difficult and uncertain. Every small success at work was proof that I could achieve something, that my life had meaning.

Despite these achievements, my inner demons didn't go away. As soon as the workday ended, the thoughts returned—that I was still far from the ideal I had once envisioned. To distract myself from these thoughts, I began to meet friends more often, throw parties, and let myself relax. Alcohol and good food became not just a part of these gatherings—they became a way to forget. This whirlwind of fun and parties consumed me. Every evening became an opportunity to escape reality, to lose myself in new acquaintances and emotions. People came and went, groups changed, but I remained at the center of this joyful vortex. Each day brought something new—new faces, new conversations, new glasses of wine, and plates of food. It seemed like life had finally gained color, even if that color was fueled by alcohol and temporary pleasures.

I became the life of the party, and I liked it. I was the one people gravitated toward, the one they wanted to spend time with. I was the center of attention, and it gave me great satisfaction. People surrounded me, and they admired me not for my appearance but for who I was—fun, interesting, and responsive. I enjoyed every moment, and in this whirl of parties and gatherings, I didn't have time to think about my body. All of it became a part of my new life. It seemed like thoughts about appearance and weight dissolved in the circle of people around me. Life felt simple and carefree, though deep down, I still knew there was something I was trying to forget.

Thoughts of losing weight still returned occasionally, but they weren't as sharp as they had been before. Now I understood that workouts and exercise had become something more than a necessity—a habit that brought me pleasure. I no longer exercised to prove something to someone or to lose pounds. Physical activity became a way to relieve stress, release emotions, and recharge. I no longer saw workouts as a punishment for eating an extra piece of cake. On the contrary, every time I left the gym, I felt light and satisfied that I had done something for myself. It became a source of joy for me, and I began to appreciate this moment as part of my new life. The thoughts about weight were still there, but they no longer determined my happiness.

My new lifestyle became my norm. I worked during the day, worked out in the evening, and partied at night. This rhythm, which many would find impossible, became natural for me. I no longer thought about changing anything. Life started to feel easier. From the moment I stopped obsessing over my weight, every day was filled with energy and confidence. Now I could enjoy the process without worrying about the outcome. My body was no longer my enemy—it had become my ally.

Over time, I realized that making peace with my body was an important step. I no longer fought with myself, no longer tried to fit into others' standards. Accepting my body gave me internal freedom. Instead of wasting energy on a struggle, I started living as I was. With this acceptance came a surprising discovery: men continued to pay attention to me. Physical attractiveness was only part of what interested them. I began to realize that my charm, intellect, kindness, sincerity, and responsiveness played no less a role. This realization helped me see myself differently. I was more than just a body, and this awareness brought a new wave of confidence.

This interest from men strengthened my feeling that looks weren't everything. They valued me not just for my figure but for who I was as a person. I started to believe that everything was happening as it should. My kindness, openness, and sincerity became the qualities that attracted people to me. This gave me a new understanding that I deserved love and respect just as I was. I no longer tried to change for someone else. I became a confident woman who knew she was appreciated for her inner qualities just as much as for her outer ones.

Accepting myself brought me the peace I had been seeking for so long. My internal struggle gradually faded away. Now, when I looked in the mirror, I didn't see a collection of flaws but a whole person. I no longer felt the need to change to be better in others' eyes. I was already good enough as I was. This realization became a true liberation for me. I no longer felt obligated to meet anyone's expectations or stereotypes. Every day, I accepted myself as I was, and it brought me inner calm and satisfaction. Now I looked at my body and my life from a completely different perspective. I no longer strived for the ideal that diets, magazines, or societal standards of beauty had once imposed on me.

I lived the way I wanted to, and I liked it. Every new day was a source of joy, not another battle with myself. My body was no longer my enemy or a constant source of stress. It had become my ally, supporting me in what I was doing. I realized that true happiness doesn't come from meeting external expectations but from inner harmony and self-acceptance. I no longer needed to run anywhere or prove anything to anyone. I was already good enough, and I didn't need any external confirmation of that fact.

From that moment on, I began to build my life on different principles. I allowed myself to enjoy life, to do what brought me joy, and to surround myself with people who valued me for who I was. I no longer feared being myself, and this gave me an incredible sense of freedom. I accepted myself with all my imperfections and learned to love myself without worrying about others' opinions. This new phase of my life became a time of inner growth and transformation. I learned not only to live in peace with myself but also to enjoy the process.

Life became simpler, easier, and happier. I realized

that you can be happy without having the «perfect» body, and that the most important thing is to be in harmony with yourself and your desires. Now I knew that my worth wasn't defined by the numbers on a scale but by who I was inside—my actions, how I treated others, and how I treated myself. This awareness brought me new strength and confidence. I no longer relied on the outside world to find my place and recognition. I had found it within myself.

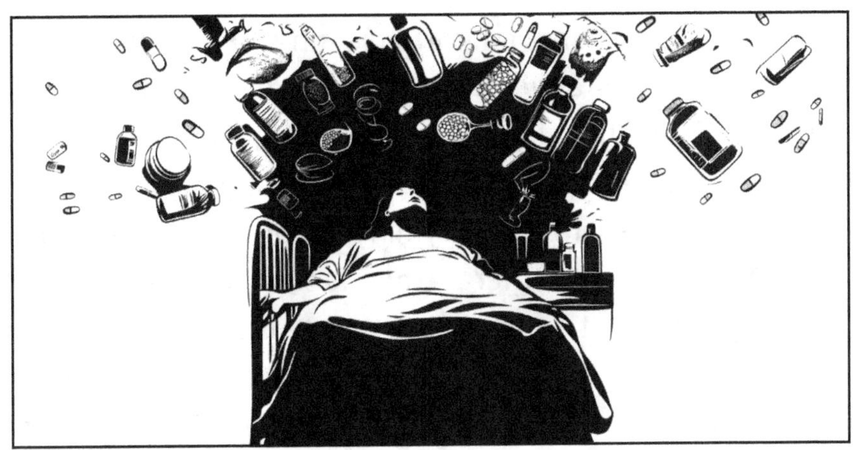

Chapter 5 — «When the Body Starts Screaming: I Can't Take It Anymore»

After gradually adapting to my new lifestyle and accepting myself internally, it felt like everything was getting simpler and easier. My confidence grew, and I started to enjoy the rhythm I had created for myself. Worries about my weight began to fade, receding into the background as if they no longer had power over me. I felt the lightness that comes when you stop constantly fighting with yourself and others' expectations. It was like being freed from shackles that had dragged me down for so long. But just when life seems manageable, fate often throws unexpected surprises.

One evening, I was getting ready for a party, confident that everything would go as usual. Drinks, food, friends, laughter—the standard night where I was the life of the party. But something felt off this time. From the start, the mood was strange, unnatural. I didn't feel the usual desire to have fun. Instead, a sense of apathy washed over me, and I couldn't explain why. Sitting at the table, I felt disconnected from everything around me, like I was there but not really there. This feeling of detachment was frightening; it reminded me that maybe I was losing control over my life. My friends noticed and asked what was wrong, but I couldn't answer them myself.

At some point, I decided that a little alcohol might help me get back to my usual state. «This is just a temporary weakness,» I convinced myself. Bourbon, which I always loved, seemed like the answer. I poured myself 1.7 ounces, certain it would lift my spirits and make the evening more enjoyable. But instead of the expected relief, things got worse with every passing minute. Rather than the familiar warmth in my body, there was a heaviness in my stomach, followed by a wave of nausea. It crept up slowly, becoming more intense with each passing moment. I thought it would pass, that it was just temporary, but it got worse until I started to vomit violently, offering no relief.

Barely making it to the bathroom, I clung to the sink, trying to alleviate my state, but the vomiting didn't stop and brought no relief. Before the vomiting started, I had taken an absorbent hoping it would halt the impending sickness. But it was all in vain. The vomiting not only didn't subside but intensified. Each new wave brought a sense of helplessness and anxiety. Weakness engulfed my entire body, my head spun, and all I could do was cling to the sink, realizing that things were spiraling out of control. At that moment, I understood that my confidence in my condition was an illusion.

Returning to my friends, I could no longer sit up; I felt so terrible. I lay down on the couch, knowing I couldn't stay among them any longer. I called a taxi and decided to go to my parents' house as I had promised to spend the night there. On the way, my condition only worsened. I was constantly nauseous, and every time the car stopped, the nausea hit with a new wave. One thought kept running through my head: What is happening to me, and when will this end? These thoughts replayed like a broken record, intensifying my fear and anxiety.

When I arrived at my parents' house, I immediately admitted how sick I felt and tried to explain my condition. My mom, as always, rushed to help me. She offered another absorbent and more water, but nothing worked. Every drop of liquid triggered another wave of vomiting. All I could do was lie there and suffer. Then the stomach pains began—so severe that I couldn't pinpoint exactly where it hurt. Everything inside me screamed in pain, and I couldn't focus on anything else. It felt like my entire world had narrowed to one endless torment. In that moment, pain became the center of my existence; nothing else mattered. After an hour and a half, I realized I couldn't take it anymore and asked my parents to call an ambulance.

The paramedics arrived quickly and acted professionally. They examined me, took my blood pressure, pulse, and temperature, and quickly realized the seriousness of the situation. They put me on a stretcher and took me to the hospital. Along the way, I tried to understand what was happening to me, what had caused this, and when it would end. I could no longer hold back my fears; each new bout of vomiting and pain drained me. My mom stayed behind while my dad came with me to support me in the hospital. When we arrived, the night doctors were ready for me. After filling out some paperwork, they took me to a room, where they hooked me up to my first IV and gave me a painkiller injection. Finally, after hours of agony, the pain began to subside, but the fear didn't go away. Lying in the hospital room, I watched the dawn through the window, thinking: What's wrong with me? That question became my only companion that night, leaving me in complete uncertainty about the future.

The next morning, the doctor came in, did a preliminary exam, and ordered some tests. A few hours later, he returned with the results. «Acute pancreatitis,» he said, without much emotion. I wasn't surprised, though I didn't fully understand what it meant. The doctor explained in detail that my lifestyle, eating habits, and alcohol consumption had led to inflammation of the pancreas. Now, I faced a long and challenging recovery. «You won't eat for the next few days. Only water and IV drips three times a day,» he added, as if this were the most common diagnosis. I knew I would have to follow his instructions, but I didn't realize how much this would change my life. In that moment, I first considered that my body might not be able to endure what I had been putting it through any longer.

I didn't understand how one could go without food entirely, but I had no choice. Since I had no appetite due to the nausea and fear, I wasn't worried about having to go without food for a long time. Every time they brought breakfast, lunch, or dinner, I looked at the food indifferently and refused. Strangely, I wasn't tormented by hunger, and the sensation of being hungry never came. With each passing day, I grew more accustomed to this state. My roommates ate their meals, but it didn't bother me at all. My body seemed to accept the lack of food, and I began to feel that I could go a long time without it and still feel relatively okay. It was a strange feeling—to live in this state, as if on autopilot. For the first time, I realized that food wasn't the center of my universe.

On the third day of fasting, the doctor finally said I could have breakfast. I was relieved, feeling like I was on the road to recovery. However, the breakfast turned out to be different from what I had expected: it was a simple boiled porridge without salt or butter. I cautiously took a spoonful and brought it to my mouth, as if testing how my body would react. But with each spoonful, disappointment washed over me. The taste was so bland that I didn't even want to continue eating. It didn't bring the relief I had hoped for, but I understood that this was part of the recovery process. Now, food was not a pleasure but a necessity.

After being discharged from the hospital, the doctor

gave me strict dietary recommendations. For several months, I had to completely avoid alcohol, fatty, fried, and spicy foods. Everything I ate had to be steamed or boiled. I was to stick to light meals: boiled vegetables, lean meats, and soups without spices. The doctor also warned against abruptly returning to my usual diet; I needed to gradually introduce new foods and monitor my body's reaction. When I got home, the first thing that surprised me was how loose my clothes felt. Weighing myself, I found out I had lost 18 pounds during my time in the hospital. It was shocking! But at the same time, I realized I would have to give up working out, which the doctor temporarily forbade to avoid overloading my body. The body I had been trying to control for so long suddenly began dictating its own terms, and I had to comply.

For the first couple of weeks, I strictly adhered to all the recommendations. My diet was simple but effective: boiled vegetables, lean broths, plenty of water, and small, frequent meals. Gradually, my weight continued to drop, though not as quickly as in the hospital. These small successes encouraged me to keep following the guidelines, and I began to believe that I could control my weight. However, after a few weeks, the loneliness began to weigh on me. I missed meeting up with friends and the times when I could socialize freely and enjoy life. One day, I decided that I had recovered enough to return to my normal social life. This decision marked my first step back toward what I had been trying so hard to escape.

One day, feeling well enough, I arranged to meet

friends for dinner. I tried to be careful, but the cheerful atmosphere quickly swept me away. I allowed myself a glass of wine and a small dessert. «Nothing bad will happen,» I thought, especially since I was still taking the medications the doctor had prescribed. But this was the first small mistake that led to a repetition of old habits. At first, everything went well, but as meetings with friends became more frequent, I started to deviate from my routine more often. Over time, my weight loss plateaued and then slowly started to increase. I knew I was slipping back into old habits, but I couldn't stop. And, as I feared, it ended with another attack: weakness, nausea, vomiting, pain...

This was my second attack in a few months. It all repeated: severe pain, vomiting, dizziness—as if by script. Again, the ambulance, the hospital, and ten days on a strict diet, five of which were without food. However, this time I felt different. I knew what to do and understood where this was all leading. My habit of breaking dietary rules was stronger than me. Despite all the doctors' efforts and my own promises, I ended up in the hospital again. Realizing that I was losing control was disheartening. The doctors already knew me, but each new day reminded me how difficult it was to break old habits. It felt like I was stuck in an endless cycle: a bit of relief, then back to the same problems. It was a lesson I just couldn't learn.

The third attack in a year became my toughest challenge. It was like a vicious circle I couldn't escape. Every time I thought things would be different this time, reality pulled me back into the same issues. Lying in the hospital room, I felt I was losing control not just of my body but of my life. The doctors no longer asked questions; they knew me and my case. Each time I returned to the hospital, I felt like my own worst enemy. I already knew what would happen next: IV drips, a strict diet, medications—all had become part of my new, terrible «routine.» This was the third time in a year, and I began to understand that if I didn't take control, this cycle would go on forever. I left the hospital feeling that I had to change everything now, or the next time could be even worse. But despite this, old habits and temptations took hold again.

And then, a few months later, the fourth attack happened. This became my final warning. When the doctor saw my discharge papers, he couldn't hide his irritation: «Do you want to die from this pain?» His words struck me like a slap in the face, making me realize that if I didn't stop, things could end tragically. The doctor said that in a year, I had collected a full set of discharge papers from all four hospital departments. Those words marked the point of no return. I understood that I couldn't continue like this any longer. This attack became the signal for radical changes. I realized that either I change my life now, or the consequences could be irreversible.

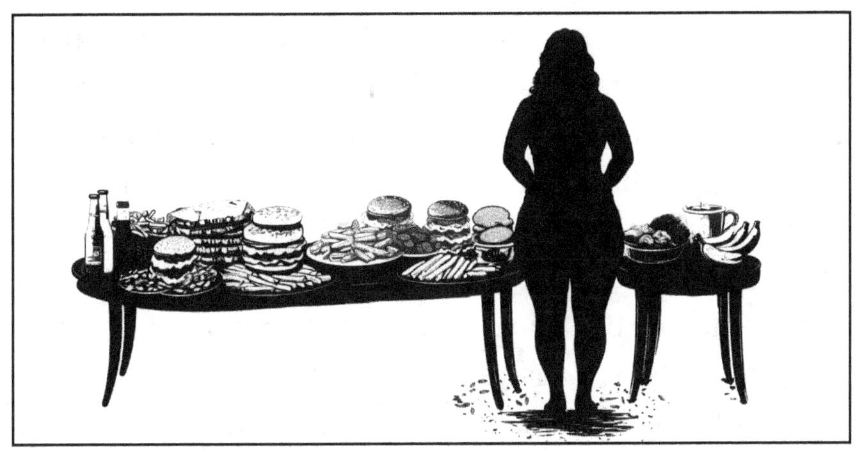

Chapter 6 — «A New Path: Letting Go of the Old and Embracing the New»

When I realized that the fourth attack of pancreatitis was my last warning, fear filled my life. It was fear for the future, fear that I would never be able to live a normal life again. The pain I felt and the doctor's words echoed in my head: «Do you want to die from this pain?» Those words were a shocking but necessary wake-up call. I knew I couldn't continue living like this. If I went back to my old habits, this cycle would never end, and next time, I might not get away with just a hospital visit. That fear became a powerful motivator for me. I faced a difficult task—not only giving up alcohol but also radically changing everything about my diet and lifestyle. It was a path full of uncertainty and doubt, but it was a path I needed to take.

Switching to a new eating regimen wasn't easy. I used to indulge my cravings without thinking about the consequences. Now, every meal became a challenge, requiring not just discipline but mindfulness. At first, it seemed almost impossible. I knew that any deviation from the recommendations could send me back to the hospital. The thought was frightening but also gave me the determination to stick to the rules. I knew that every small concession to my old cravings could cost me my life. This realization gave me the strength to follow the diet despite all the difficulties.

My main task was to completely restructure my diet, making it as easy as possible for my pancreas. The doctor repeated the same strict guidelines: eliminate everything fatty, fried, spicy, and, of course, give up alcohol. Everything I could eat had to be boiled, stewed, or steamed. One of the key elements was organizing my eating schedule: six times a day in small portions to maintain an even load on my digestive system. It sounded complicated, but I was determined to try. In this new regimen, I needed to find a balance between healthiness and taste, so I wouldn't perceive my diet as a punishment but rather as a way of self-care.

Each day started with breakfast. It was oatmeal cooked in water, to which I added a boiled egg and a bit of Greek yogurt. The breakfast was simple but nutritious and healthy. It became more than just a meal—it was a symbol of a new beginning. A couple of hours later came the second breakfast—usually a light snack: cottage cheese with yogurt or some dry biscuits. I could also have half a banana or a baked apple. Lunch consisted of a light soup made with vegetable broth and some lean chicken fillet. As a side dish, I chose buckwheat or rice, with portions being about 3–4 tablespoons. Sometimes, to diversify the diet, I made a puree of pumpkin and zucchini—their mild taste paired nicely with boiled chicken. This regimen became a ritual that helped me feel in control of my body.

For an afternoon snack, I picked something light: yogurt or a baked apple. Sometimes, when I craved something sweet, I allowed myself bananas or baby food. Sweets were strictly forbidden, so the only exception was dry biscuits and baked fruits, which did not irritate my stomach and pancreas. Dinner was even lighter—boiled fish or steamed chicken cutlets with some stewed vegetables. Everything was cooked in small quantities, with portions around 150 grams. I decided not to buy ready-made meals and only eat freshly prepared food—what was cooked on that very day. In rare cases, when I couldn't cook, I would eat a serving of plain baby food. Introducing these rules into my life was a challenge but also an opportunity to learn to care for myself in a new way.

The key to success with this diet was paying close attention to portion sizes and the quality of the food. Every bite mattered. Eating became not just a diet but an important ritual of self-care. Despite the limitations, I learned to enjoy simple dishes and even found pleasure in them. Gradually, I began to see how my relationship with food was changing. Food used to be a way to satisfy hunger or stress, but now it was an act of self-love and care for my body.

Portion size became a crucial factor in my new eating regimen. I got used to eating smaller, more frequent meals—five to six times a day instead of three large meals. For example, my morning portion of oatmeal was about 150 grams, approximately 3–4 tablespoons. It was enough to fill me up but not overwhelm my stomach. Lunch was also prepared in small amounts—a serving of soup was around 200 milliliters, about half a standard bowl. Side dishes like buckwheat or rice were measured at 100–120 grams to avoid overeating.

For dinner, I preferred something light. Steamed chicken fillet, baked fish, or vegetable stew became my favorite dishes. A portion of fish was about 100–120 grams, which was enough to make me feel full but not overloaded. When I wanted something light and simple, I made a vegetable puree from pumpkin and carrots—one of the most pleasant side dishes I discovered. The puree was easy to make, and a 150-gram portion filled the plate halfway, creating the feeling of a complete meal. This was a learning process: I discovered which foods and in what quantities worked for my body's benefit.

Giving up alcohol entirely was another crucial part of my new lifestyle. I understood that alcohol, in any form, even in minimal doses, could trigger a new attack, which I couldn't afford. Every time I was offered a drink at gatherings or celebrations, I calmly declined. The fear of ending up in the hospital was stronger than any temptation. I no longer saw alcohol as an integral part of social life. On the contrary, the realization that health is more important than temporary pleasure made it easy to refuse. This refusal became a kind of act of self-respect, a statement that my health and well-being were a priority.

Initially, it wasn't easy, but over time I realized that my new diet not only helped manage my digestive issues but also contributed to gradual weight loss. My weight began to decrease steadily, and this gave me real satisfaction. Every lost pound was not just a number on the scale but proof that I was taking the right steps. This process wasn't fast, but I saw the results, and it inspired me to keep going. Gradually, food stopped being an enemy. It became my way of caring for myself, showing love for my body and respect for my efforts.

The diet, which initially seemed like a difficult and boring necessity, started bringing me joy. I learned to enjoy simple dishes, finding a balance of taste and benefit. Food was no longer an enemy, and I no longer felt internal tension before every meal. On the contrary, it became my way of caring for my body and feeling healthy and energetic. I realized that caring for my nutrition was not a punishment but an opportunity to show love and respect for myself.

At the same time, I also figured out how to handle social situations. Over time, I learned to say «no» to offers to drink or try something «unhealthy.» At gatherings, I started bringing my own food and calmly explained that it was better for my health. My friends accepted my new habits and even started asking what they could prepare for me so I could join in the meals. Their care and understanding became very important to me; it helped me not feel isolated or deprived of the usual joys of life. This was a huge step in accepting myself and my new lifestyle.

The new eating regimen and mindful attitude towards food not only resolved my digestive issues but also promoted gradual and steady weight loss. This gave me not only physical relief but also psychological satisfaction. Seeing the positive changes in my body, I felt I was heading in the right direction, and it motivated me to keep taking care of myself. Now, every meal was not just a dietary requirement but a small victory on the path to a new, healthier, and happier life.

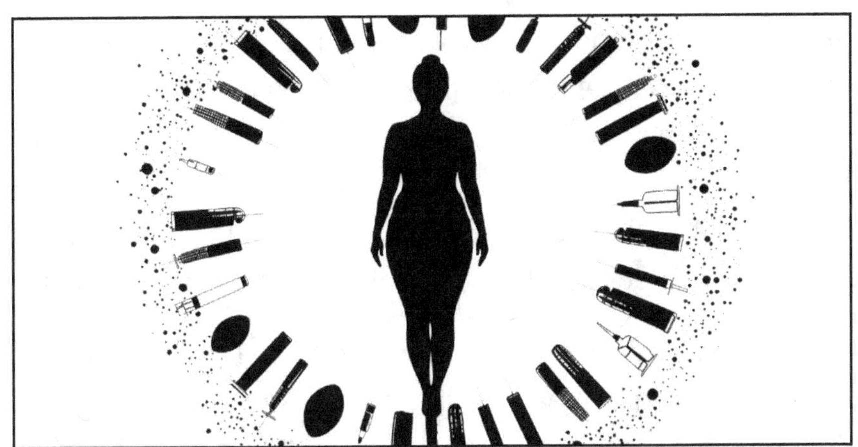

Chapter 7 — «When You're a Frequent Visitor to the Emergency Room»

After I thought I had tackled pancreatitis and learned to live with my new eating habits, it seemed like I could finally relax and enjoy life. Deep inside, I felt victorious—I had been through so much, learned to control my diet, and managed to avoid temptations that could harm my health. But despite all my efforts, my body kept sending warning signals. One such signal was high blood pressure that just wouldn't go down. For a long time, I couldn't figure out why it stayed so high. Instead of addressing the issue and finding its root cause, I chose to turn a blind eye. I kept telling myself it was temporary and that, eventually, my blood pressure would stabilize on its own. I neither had the time nor the desire to run from doctor to doctor for more tests. I was already exhausted from endless medical examinations and wanted to push these thoughts aside. As long as my blood pressure didn't cause any serious discomfort, I decided not to worry about it and put off finding a solution. It felt like I had finally found a balance where I could maintain my health at an acceptable level without unnecessary stress.

However, as it often happens, the body had its own way of reminding me that I couldn't keep ignoring problems. One day, on my way to visit my parents, I suddenly felt a sharp pain in my back. It was so unexpected and intense that I could barely sit in the car, and with each passing minute, it grew more unbearable. At first, I thought it might be a relapse of pancreatitis, having experienced similar symptoms before, but this time, things were different. The pain wasn't accompanied by nausea, and it seemed to be in a completely different location. Stopping at a pharmacy along the way, I bought a painkiller, hoping it would help me make it home. When I finally reached my parents' place, I lay down to rest, hoping a short nap would make me feel better. After an hour of sleep, the pain did start to subside, and I convinced myself that it was probably just a case of overexertion. I didn't give it much thought at that moment and tried to forget about what had happened, hoping it was just a one-off incident brought on by stress or fatigue.

But the peace was short-lived. A few days later, I woke up early in the morning feeling fantastic. The day promised to be productive, I was in a great mood, and the weather outside was beautiful and sunny. I had a lot of plans, including several important online meetings. I prepared my breakfast as usual—oatmeal with a boiled egg and green tea, my faithful companions in healthy eating. But before I could finish my tea, I suddenly started to feel a severe decline in my condition. I began to shake, my skin was covered with goosebumps, and I felt a chill even though the room was warm. Soon, the chills were joined by a sharp, cramping pain in my lower back that grew stronger by the minute. At first, I tried to stay calm, thinking it might just be a temporary ailment, and decided to lie down for a while. However, it quickly became clear that the pain was not going away, but instead, it was intensifying. Panic set in.

I had no idea what was happening to my body. Waves of pain washed over me, each spasm feeling more intense than the last. I realized I couldn't wait any longer and, despite my fear, decided to call an ambulance. My past experiences with doctors and hospitals had taught me not to take any medications before an examination, so as not to distort the clinical picture. While explaining my situation to the dispatcher, my vision began to blur from the pain. I warned them that I might lose consciousness and that I would leave the door open so the paramedics could come in without obstacles. The pain was relentless, and it felt like my condition was worsening by the minute. I couldn't sit; I couldn't lie down—the pain was so severe that I was pacing around my apartment like a trapped animal, searching for any position that might bring me some relief.

When the paramedics arrived, I could barely speak

but managed to describe my symptoms. They quickly examined me, and within a few minutes, the doctor delivered the diagnosis: kidney stones. I couldn't believe my ears. Kidney stones? I had never heard of this diagnosis before and had no idea how it was connected to what I was feeling. The paramedics explained that I probably had a stone in my kidney, which was causing the attack. I was in shock. How was that possible? I had been eating right, avoiding alcohol, and taking care of my health. It all seemed like some bizarre coincidence. As I struggled to comprehend what they were saying, the medics gave me a painkiller injection, and the pain began to fade. I had started to think about declining hospitalization, but the paramedics strongly advised against it. They explained that the situation needed to be monitored and that it was better to undergo all necessary examinations now.

Arriving at the hospital, I felt devastated. How could this happen again? After all my efforts, I was back in the emergency room, going through the familiar routine of registration, tests, and doctor exams. Inside, a mix of frustration and despair bubbled up. The diagnosis confirmed by the hospital doctor seemed like a misunderstanding. I couldn't believe that I actually had a kidney stone and that this would once again require serious treatment. The next day, they performed a CT scan, and I saw the accursed stone on the screen, looking like a foreign object stuck inside my body. When the doctor explained that the stone was large and needed to be removed, I felt sheer horror. Surgery—that was the last thing I wanted, especially after everything I had already been through.

I couldn't believe I was back in this situation. The thought of an impending surgery literally paralyzed me. I asked for time to think, even though I knew deep down that I likely had no choice. The doctor explained that the stone was too large and that no medications would help anymore. However, he prescribed a temporary treatment to alleviate my condition and gave me a few days to ponder my options. At that moment, as soon as I stepped out of the doctor's office, my legs gave way. Right there in the hospital corridor, in front of everyone, I fainted. When I came to, there were nurses and doctors around me, and I smelled the strong scent of ammonia. The doctor stood by my side with a smile and said, «You're such a scaredy-cat!» I tried to smile back, even though my mind was in complete chaos. I had no idea how I was going to cope with yet another blow from fate.

Returning home, I felt shattered. It seemed like the whole world had collapsed on my shoulders. I began seeking other opinions, hoping to find some glimmer of hope to avoid surgery. I visited several other clinics, consulted different specialists, but they all said the same thing: surgery was inevitable. Each new doctor visit brought growing disappointment. I couldn't believe I was back in this position. Nearly losing hope, I met an acquaintance who told me about a doctor who had helped his parents avoid surgery. I clung to this opportunity like a lifeline and immediately scheduled an appointment.

During the consultation, the doctor thoroughly examined my tests and confirmed that the situation was serious. However, he suggested trying alternative treatment with homeopathic remedies that, according to him, could dissolve kidney stones. He warned me upfront that there were no guarantees and that I had a very dense stone that might not respond to treatment. But I agreed to this experiment because I couldn't reconcile myself to the idea of surgery. The doctor prescribed me a course of medication and an even stricter diet. I had to eliminate all meat and fish broths, as well as greens like spinach and watercress, which could contribute to stone formation. This time, the dietary restrictions didn't cause me despair. I was already used to my limited diet and saw this as another step toward recovery.

For six months, I adhered to a strict diet and took the medications, hoping that the treatment would work and I could avoid surgery. I gave up many familiar foods, eating only those that were as safe as possible for my kidneys. It was oatmeal cooked in water, steamed vegetables, boiled meat, and fish prepared without salt and spices. From the greens, I only kept dill and parsley, and even then, in very small amounts. I practically eliminated all heavy food, following the doctor's recommendations. I didn't feel much discomfort since I was already used to the restrictions and viewed them as a necessity. Besides, I noticed improvements in my general condition: the pain became less frequent, and I started to hope that the treatment was working. Every day I carefully monitored my well-being and tried not to miss taking my medications.

However, after these six months, the doctor reviewed all my tests and said that, unfortunately, there were hardly any changes in my condition. The stone, if it had shrunk, had done so by an insignificant percentage that didn't save me from surgery. My heart sank. I was crushed and disappointed. Everything I had done seemed pointless. Despite all my discipline and efforts, I found myself once again on the brink of the operating table. The doctor gently but firmly made it clear that there was no more time to waste and that I needed to prepare for surgery. This time, I didn't faint, but my emotions were on edge. Thousands of questions spun in my mind: Why? I had worked so hard, taken care of myself, eaten properly. Why again? But there were no answers. All I could do was accept the situation and prepare for what lay ahead.

Three weeks later, I had a planned surgery to remove the stone. It was a rather complex procedure, but the doctors managed it successfully. A week after the surgery, I was discharged from the hospital and went home with a new set of recommendations. Only then, as I left the hospital, did they explain to me that, in addition to my tendency to form stones, I also had another problem—I wasn't drinking enough fluids. It turned out that my body lacked water, and because of this, the minerals from the food and liquid I consumed were settling in my kidneys, forming stones. This was a revelation to me. Additionally, the quality of the water I was drinking had also played a role. My body couldn't handle mineralized water, which worsened the situation.

The doctor explained that the stone they removed had been forming for many years. It had been the cause of my high blood pressure and elevated temperature that had plagued me for several years. Only when I began to lose weight did my kidney shift slightly, triggering the stone's movement and causing all the symptoms I experienced. The doctor warned me that monitoring my kidneys' condition would now be a constant part of my life and that regular check-ups would help prevent the problem from recurring. I had to accept that these visits would become part of my routine.

Leaving the hospital, I tried to make sense of everything that had happened. My body was not just a complex mechanism but a whole set of factors, each of which influenced my health. I was struck by how long the stone had been forming in my body and how it was connected to my blood pressure and other symptoms. All those years, I had been battling various problems without realizing they were linked. Now I understood that my health required not just control but full attention and care. I couldn't afford to treat my body carelessly anymore. I realized that even the smallest changes in lifestyle could have serious consequences, and this made me reassess my habits once again.

Five and a half months after the surgery, I started preparing for a routine check-up. But one morning, upon waking up, I felt a familiar chill and shiver coursing through my body. Abdominal pain hit me with new force, and I couldn't believe it was happening again. Inside, anger bubbled up. How was this possible? I had done everything right, followed all the recommendations, and drank the required amount of water. At that moment, I recalled the doctor's words about my body's tendency to form stones. This was the reality I would have to live with, but I couldn't accept that it had happened so soon. This time, I didn't panic like before. I felt only anger and disappointment.

Remembering what the doctor had said about my body's propensity for stone formation, I realized that this was indeed part of my life, something I couldn't escape. I called an ambulance, understanding that I needed to act quickly. As soon as I was in the hospital, they ran tests again, and the doctor confirmed the worst: another stone had formed. This one was smaller and less dense, but it didn't change the situation. Despite all my efforts, my body continued to create problems. It was like a vicious cycle with no way out. The doctor explained that this time the surgery would not be as complicated and suggested performing it within the next few hours to avoid delays. I felt like the ground was slipping from under my feet. Just six months ago, I had gone through this, and here I was again. My mind couldn't process what was happening, and my body was already preparing for another ordeal. The doctor was so certain of the need for surgery that I couldn't argue with him.

I barely had time to process what was happening before they sent me for pre-operative procedures. I didn't have time to think, which was probably for the best, as otherwise, I might have panicked again. Forty minutes later, I was already lying in the operating room, where they performed an epidural anesthesia, and I remained conscious throughout the procedure. The doctor joked and chatted with me as he removed the stone naturally. Although the situation was serious, his calmness and confidence helped me stay composed. Unlike the first surgery, this one felt more routine, leaving me in a mix of bewilderment and acceptance. It all went quickly, and a few hours later, I was resting in my room. I felt relieved, though inside, there was still anger at the situation. It seemed that no matter what I did, every moment could bring a new surprise. But despite this, I realized that I was still fighting and could cope with this too.

Returning home after the second surgery, I felt a swirl of emotions. On one hand, I was grateful to the doctors for their help, for the successful operation without complications. On the other hand, I felt a sense of despair. Despite all my efforts, I couldn't fully control my health. Even the strictest diets and rejection of harmful habits couldn't guarantee that I wouldn't face new problems. This was a tough lesson for me. I realized that some things can't be controlled 100%, and that's probably the hardest part of accepting myself and my body.

After these two surgeries, endless doctor visits, and constant health monitoring, I began to understand that life was teaching me humility and acceptance. No matter how hard I tried to control everything, no matter how many efforts I made, some things simply can't be controlled. The body is a complex system that sometimes behaves contrary to all our efforts and plans. I realized that it's not only important to care for my body but also to accept it as it is, with all its flaws and peculiarities. Humility doesn't mean giving up the fight. Humility is the ability to understand that not everything is in our hands, and that's okay. Life constantly teaches us lessons, and each one holds its own wisdom.

In the end, I learned to live with this knowledge. I no longer strive to control everything that happens to my body completely. I accept it as it is and understand that in this acceptance lies my strength. Each new day is an opportunity to learn something new about myself, my health, and life in general. I no longer fear my health problems because I know they are part of my journey. Humility and acceptance do not make me weaker. On the contrary, they make me stronger because I learn to live in harmony with myself, not in constant struggle with what I can't change. And although there may be new challenges ahead, I am ready to face them, knowing that, in the end, things will turn out the way they should. Now, I don't try to control everything but do my best to guide and maintain my condition at the proper level.

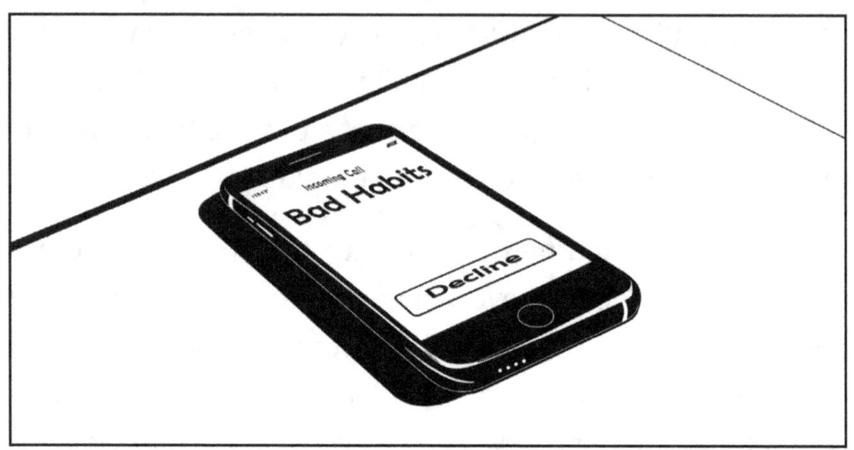

Chapter 8 — «Breaking the Habit Cycle and Starting Fresh»

As I mentioned earlier, for many years I tried to change. I tried different diets, temporarily gave up alcohol, exercised, but I always ended up falling back. It seemed like these were just small setbacks along my path, not requiring deep reflection. However, I didn't realize that my old habits were so deeply ingrained that I needed a radical intervention to break out of this cycle. And then, after my fourth visit to the emergency room's surgery department, I finally understood that I could no longer put off making changes. This was no longer a coincidence; it was a pattern I had created through my decisions and lifestyle.

Each flare-up of my illness became another link in the chain of events I stubbornly built, sinking deeper into my comfort zone. At that moment, there was no fear—there was awareness. It wasn't panic but a quiet, firm understanding that everything depended solely on me and my decisions. I was standing on the edge, and only I could change the direction of my life.

The decision to give up socializing with friends seemed radical, but it was a necessary step. My social circle, with whom I spent most of my time, was closely tied to bad habits—alcohol, high-calorie food, late-night parties. I understood that every time I met with them, I risked slipping up—having an extra glass of wine, eating something fried or sweet. These gatherings were a kind of trap that pulled me backward. I decided to temporarily isolate myself from such influences, reducing communication to phone calls. It was a tough test for me, but also a test of how ready I was to give up old habits for the sake of my health.

Over time, I realized that this isolation gave me the necessary space to focus on myself and my needs. During this period, I rethought my priorities and reassessed my relationships with those around me. It turned out that by stepping back from external influences, I was able to hear my true desires and aspirations, which became the starting point for my recovery.

Practical advice: If you feel that your environment negatively influences you, don't be afraid to temporarily step away from familiar social connections. It doesn't mean you're losing friends; it means you're putting your health first. Replacing

physical meetings with phone calls or online communication can help you stay connected without external pressure.

The next step was completely giving up alcohol and unhealthy food. This was not just following the doctors' advice—it was my conscious decision. I realized that every glass of wine or serving of fried food was causing irreparable harm to my body. I removed all fatty, fried, smoked, and preserved foods from my diet. Initially, it seemed like an extreme restriction, as I was used to rich flavors and a variety of dishes. However, over time, I realized these changes were vital. I started replacing my usual meals with simpler ones, using minimal spices and seasonings. Only basic spices and Greek yogurt instead of sauces, which had previously filled my dishes, remained.

At first, it was like traveling into the unknown—new flavors and textures I wasn't ready for. But gradually, I learned to enjoy the lightness of food, and each day my body became more responsive to such changes. New dishes became a symbol of a new stage in my life, a stage where I chose to take care of myself.

Practical advice: Start replacing heavy and fatty sauces with lighter options, such as Greek yogurt or light dressings based on olive oil. Experiment with simple spices and fresh herbs—this allows you to maintain the taste of your dishes without excess calories and overload for your body.

One of the most challenging tasks was giving up sweets. For many years, sweets had been my comfort, especially in moments of stress or fatigue. Sugar was my drug, and the idea of giving it up entirely seemed impossible. But I knew that without this step, I wouldn't be able to change my life. Instead of completely depriving myself of joy, I decided to replace sweets with fruit. Bananas and apples became my main allies in the fight against my sugar addiction. It was a tough path, requiring a lot of willpower. However, over time, I realized that it's possible to enjoy natural products without harming your health.

Sugar consumption dropped sharply, and I felt my cravings for sweets decrease. This process wasn't immediate—it was a gradual reprogramming of my body and mindset. I learned to find joy in other things, and sweets ceased to be my primary source of pleasure.

Practical advice: If you find it difficult to give up sweets, try replacing them with fruit. Choose those that satisfy your sweet cravings but contain natural sugars and beneficial vitamins. Gradually reduce the amount of sugar in your diet, and you'll notice how your body stops craving it in large amounts.

An important step in my transformation was giving up pork. Pork had always been part of my diet, but its fat content no longer suited my body. With the shift to lighter eating, I replaced pork with chicken and turkey—light, lean meats that provided me with necessary protein without overloading my digestive system. Fish also became part of my diet, though I cooked it only once or twice a week. But the key change was the way I prepared food. Now, everything was steamed, boiled, or stewed. Frying, even in minimal oil, became taboo. Even the oven was out of use for a while to avoid the temptation of using seasonings and oils that increased appetite.

Practical advice: Try cooking dishes by steaming or stewing them—it not only preserves more nutrients but also helps avoid adding extra fats. Invest in a quality steamer or slow cooker—they will greatly simplify the cooking process and help you stick to healthy eating.

Another crucial step was starting to eat in small portions. This wasn't just a medical recommendation—it was my strategy to restore the normal size of my stomach. After years of overeating, my stomach was stretched, and I needed to relearn how to feel full. Small portions became a key element of this process. I began eating not only less but also more frequently—up to 6 times a day. This helped me maintain energy levels and avoid overeating.

I learned to savor every bite of food, instead of devouring it in a hurry. This was a new experience—enjoying food, not consuming it to fill an inner void. I discovered that even a small portion of food could bring satisfaction when eaten mindfully.

Practical advice: Start using small plates to control portion sizes. Drink water before eating to partially fill your stomach, and try to eat slowly—this will help you feel fuller and avoid overeating.

The first two months after these changes were incredibly difficult. My brain was desperately resisting the new regime, and every morning began with the thought of how to return to old habits. I dreamed about familiar food, about the tastes I loved so much. It seemed that every small portion was not enough, that I was constantly hungry. However, this was only a temporary phenomenon. I understood that even an extra spoonful of oatmeal could send me back to the hospital. This fear was a powerful motivator to keep fighting.

I realized that every little victory in resisting the temptation to eat something unhealthy brought me closer to my goal. It was a process of mental restructuring, where I was learning to live anew, shedding old destructive habits. Each day, I noticed that the craving for old tastes was weakening, and with it came a new understanding and acceptance of myself.

Practical advice: In the first months of change, be prepared for your brain to resist the new regime. This is normal. To overcome this, find replacements for your habits—for example, instead of seeking comfort in food, find other sources of joy and support: reading, walking, socializing.

Joy didn't come immediately, but when the weight began to drop, I felt real relief. It became confirmation that I was on the right path. I no longer felt constantly hungry—on the contrary, I started enjoying the process of healthy eating. My schedule—5-6 times a day—became part of my new lifestyle, and I stopped thinking about food obsessively.

However, those around me thought differently. My mom even joked that I was eating constantly, but in reality, I was sticking to strict control. This control gave me a sense of power over myself and my habits. I was no longer a slave to food—I became the master of my diet.

Practical advice: Create a clear meal schedule for yourself. Frequent but small meals help maintain energy levels and avoid feelings of hunger. Prepare a set of healthy snacks in advance to avoid slipping into unhealthy eating.

To take full control of my diet, I started weighing my food and counting calories. It turned out to be much simpler than I initially thought. At first, I assumed it would be tedious, but soon it became a regular practice for me. Buying kitchen scales turned out to be a very helpful decision, as I began to realize how much I was consuming each day.

My limit was 1500 calories—a recommendation doctors had given me back in 2009. If breakfast was close to 600 calories, I knew that I didn't have much left for the rest of the day. This control helped me avoid overeating and taught me to plan my meals more mindfully. I became more attentive to my diet, to what I ate and in what quantity.

Weighing food became a kind of ritual that helped me stay within my goal. It no longer seemed burdensome—on the contrary, I found a certain joy in it. With each passing day, I learned to better understand my body, its needs, and its capabilities.

Practical advice: If you start counting calories, begin by recording everything you eat. Use an app or just a notebook to track your diet. Weigh your food—it will help you control the number of calories you consume and maintain balance.

Gradually, I began to notice how my attitude toward food and life was changing. Strict control over portions and calories became not something stressful but a natural part of my day. Each day, I felt lighter—not only physically but also emotionally. I stopped justifying every portion I ate, and instead, I found confidence in my decisions and actions. This process of transformation was slow, but it proved to be incredibly beneficial for my physical and emotional well-being.

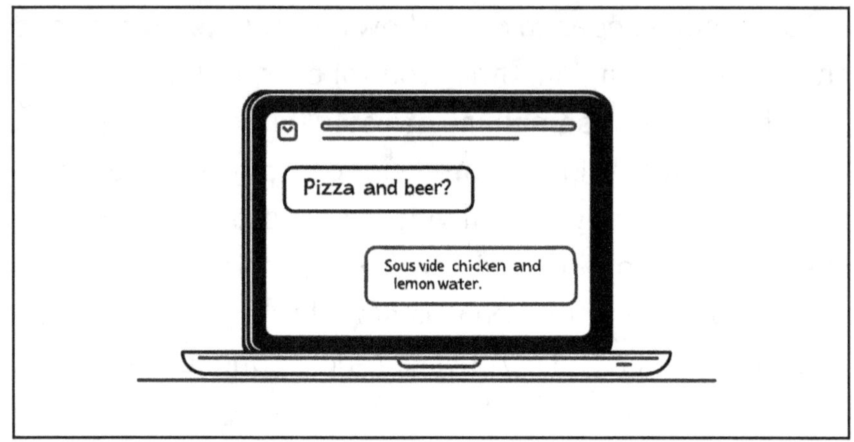

Chapter 9 — «How My New Habits Changed My Social Life»

After two months of isolating myself from society, I began to realize that I didn't need other people's approval to make decisions. Before, I used to think that other people's opinions played a big role in my life, and I often sought their support. However, being alone and cutting myself off from external influences made me understand that my independence and self-sufficiency were key elements of my new lifestyle. There was something liberating in this realization: I no longer relied on other people's advice or opinions. Now I could hear my own voice, which had become my main guide. It gave me a sense of freedom and confidence, knowing that all my decisions were my conscious choice and not a result of someone else's expectations.

During this time, I learned to trust myself more than ever before. Being alone with my thoughts, I realized that true freedom comes when you stop seeking external approval. It was a kind of rebirth. I realized that my worth wasn't measured by other people's opinions, and this understanding allowed me to see life from a new perspective.

However, I didn't want to isolate myself from society completely. Living outside of the social circle was never part of my plan—it was important to remain a part of my social environment, but without falling back into harmful habits. I needed to find a balance between maintaining a healthy lifestyle and returning to social life, where old habits like drinking and unhealthy eating could tempt me again. Re-entering society became a kind of test for me. I accepted the challenge, but with a new understanding: to avoid falling back into old habits, I developed clear rules that helped me stay in control. I now knew that my health was more important than any social rituals.

This process wasn't easy. Social pressure and the fear of judgment from others were constant challenges. However, when faced with it head-on, I realized that my choices were mine alone. I created my own set of rules and principles that allowed me to stay true to myself, even when surrounded by those who still followed their old habits.

Practical advice: If you're returning to a group of friends or colleagues where you might face temptations, plan your actions ahead of time. Prepare mentally and come up with

I decided to stick to a simple but proven principle: if I was going to an event where there would be food, I would bring something with me. It could be a small snack that wouldn't raise any questions from others but would keep me in control of what I was eating. This turned out to be very effective—I didn't need to search for suitable food, and I knew I could stay within my nutrition plan. If the event was such that bringing food was inappropriate, I would plan ahead to eat fruits—there's always at least a few options at any buffet. I tried to calculate in advance how much I could eat without breaking my regimen. And if there were no suitable dishes at all, I would simply smile and say, «I'm not hungry, thanks.» This became my universal answer, allowing me to politely avoid unnecessary explanations.

Practical advice: Always plan ahead. If you're attending an event with food, find out in advance what will be offered or bring a healthy snack with you. This will help you stick to your decisions and avoid uncomfortable situations where you have nothing to eat. Preparation is key, especially when you're just starting your journey to change your habits.

I placed my health and well-being as my top priority. This became my new life principle: if something or someone tried to throw me off track, I would simply remind myself that my goal was more important. In the past, I might have caved under pressure, trying not to stand out or cause discomfort, but now I learned to be independent in my decisions. It required inner strength and confidence that my path was the right one. If someone didn't like that I wasn't eating or drinking like they were, it wasn't my problem. It was their insecurities and issues that they were projecting onto me. Before, I would have worried about it, but now I understood that I couldn't let others influence my personal choices. My health and my goals would always come first.

Practical advice: Don't be afraid to put your priorities first. This is not selfishness but an act of self-care. Learn to calmly and confidently stand by your decisions without feeling guilty. Confidence in your actions is key to staying on track, despite the influence of others.

People who are «genuinely concerned» that I'm not enjoying the food or who try to find a way for me to drink alcohol with them aren't really doing it for my sake, but for theirs. This was an important realization I had while observing the reactions of those around me. They might feel uncomfortable being around someone who doesn't drink or eat the same things they do, and it had nothing to do with my choices. When a person can't control their desires and doesn't want to take responsibility for their decisions, they try to shift the blame onto others. So, these people may feel insecure and want everyone around them to act just like they do. I realized that it all came down to their internal issues and anxieties, and it no longer concerned me.

This was a moment of enlightenment for me. I understood that my refusal to conform to other people's expectations wasn't a sign of disrespect towards them but rather a demonstration of respect for myself. This understanding helped me to calmly take my stand and not let other people's insecurities influence my decisions.

Practical advice: If you feel pressure from others trying to get you to act in a way that suits them, just remember: these are their issues, not yours. Don't take on other people's insecurities, and don't let them influence your decisions. Be confident in your actions and know that your path is your personal choice, and no one can make you stray from it.

Over time, my friends became so accustomed to my new eating habits and refusal to drink alcohol that they began not only to accept it as normal but also to genuinely inquire about what I was doing to achieve such results. Their questions became more frequent, and they wanted to know how I had managed to so radically change my life. Although not everyone followed my advice, most showed genuine interest in my approach. Moreover, some friends, who truly cared about my comfort, started asking in advance what I could eat from what was planned at the event. If there was nothing suitable, they would offer to prepare something specifically for me so that I wouldn't have to worry about it. This was a real sign of respect and support from them, and I felt that my efforts were finally paying off not only for me but also for those around me.

This moment was special for me. I realized that my decision to change my lifestyle didn't just affect me but also touched my surroundings. It was a sign that my new habits were starting to bring positive changes not only in my life but also in the lives of those around me.

Practical advice: Be open with your friends and loved ones about your needs. Those who genuinely value your efforts and care for you will definitely support you. Don't hesitate to discuss the menu of events in advance to avoid awkward situations, and be ready to offer alternative dishes. This will help you feel comfortable and avoid unnecessary stress.

I realized that my position, despite the pressure from others, was more stable than theirs. I was confident in my choice and knew that my refusal to drink alcohol or eat unhealthy food made me stronger, while they continued to seek comfort in habits that were destroying their health. Every time I refused alcohol or sweets at a party, it strengthened my confidence and determination. I no longer needed other people's approval or understanding. My health, my progress, and my determination had become more important than any opinion. With each refusal, I grew stronger, and it gave me an inner peace that I had never known before.

Practical advice: Strengthen your resolve with every refusal of old habits. Every time you stand by your decisions, you become stronger and more confident. Over time, this becomes your natural state, and you no longer need to explain yourself to others. Your confidence in yourself will only grow.

With each refusal, I learned to trust myself more. I stopped fearing the reactions of those around me and started listening more to my inner voice. It didn't matter anymore what others thought of me, because I knew I was doing it for myself and not for anyone else. Others might not understand or accept my choice, but that no longer influenced my decisions. My health became my top priority, and this inner balance made me even stronger. Every step towards self-control and awareness brought me closer to new levels of confidence and independence.

I realized that within us is an enormous reservoir of strength and determination that we often underestimate. My new lifestyle became a kind of school for me, where every day I learned to strengthen my willpower and develop my awareness.

Practical advice: Listen to your inner voice and follow it, even if it goes against the expectations of others. Your health and well-being are more important than anyone else's opinion. Listen to yourself, and you'll be stronger in resisting external pressure.

Over time, my friends stopped trying to persuade me to drink or eat something unhealthy. They got used to my new lifestyle, and although some initially laughed at my refusals, they eventually began to respect my determination. This process took time, but it proved to me that if you're consistent and confident in your choice, people around you will eventually begin to see it as normal. I learned that willpower and patience are key components of success.

Now, looking back, I understood that I had gone through an important stage, where not only had I changed, but my surroundings had also learned to respect my decisions.

This was a real test for me—learning to stand up for my priorities and beliefs in a society that didn't always support my aspirations. But with each day, I became more confident in my choice and saw how gradually the attitude of others towards me changed.

Practical advice: If people don't understand or laugh at your choice at first, it's normal. Just keep following your principles, and sooner or later they'll get used to it. It's important to be consistent and confident in yourself. Over time, people will start to respect your efforts and see you as an example of resilience and confidence.

In the end, I realized that my health, my goals, and my well-being are my responsibility. No one else is responsible for what I eat or drink, and no one can make me stray from my principles. I began to understand that putting myself first isn't selfish, but a necessity for my well-being. I no longer felt obligated to conform to those around me, and this realization brought me incredible relief. I found peace and tranquility in my new approach to life, and it was one of the best discoveries on my journey to health.

This was a moment of true freedom. Freedom from other people's expectations, judgments, and pressure. I learned to live as I saw fit, and it brought me inner harmony and confidence. My health became my priority, and I'm proud of how far I've come.

Practical advice: Learn to put yourself first. This will help you maintain confidence and resist external pressure. Your goals and health are more important than public opinion. Others may not immediately understand your choice, but over time, you'll feel freer and stronger if you stick to your priorities.

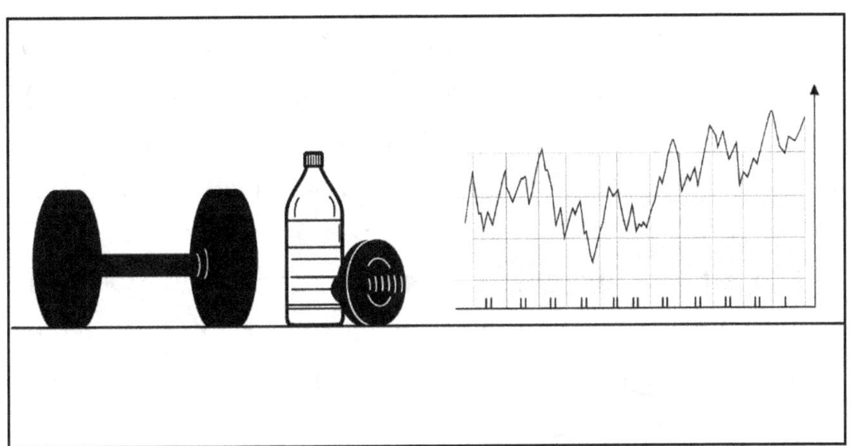

Chapter 10 — «How Exercise Helped Complete My Recovery»

In May 2021, I realized it was time to reintroduce exercise into my life, despite the challenges that arose after the surgeries. My feelings were mixed: on one hand, I feared potential complications, but on the other, I longed to return to an active life, to feel that energy and strength again. After losing a significant amount of weight and recovering my health, I came to understand that maintaining physical fitness wasn't just a phase but a necessity for a fulfilling life. As I started losing weight, every pound I shed made it easier to perform exercises that once seemed impossible. However, I also understood that along with the fat, I was losing muscle, and muscle was essential for me to feel strong and energetic. I didn't just want to lose weight; I wanted to strengthen my body and take care of my skin, which, I knew, needed tightening and recovery. But due to my kidney stone removal surgery, I was prohibited from engaging in overly intense physical activities. This became a challenge: I was eager for results, yet I had to strictly follow my doctor's recommendations and be mindful of my health. This internal conflict between desire and caution became a new aspect of my journey.

Practical advice: After serious medical procedures, it is always important to consult with a doctor and a fitness specialist before returning to physical activity. Start with light exercises and take it slow. Steady, gradual progress will help you avoid complications while building strength without overloading your body.

I decided to approach my recovery wisely: I bought a smart scale to track my progress and scheduled a consultation with my trainer, whom I had worked with before I started going in and out of hospitals. When I returned to him after 2.5 years, his reaction was priceless. He stared at me for a long time as if he didn't recognize me, and then his jaw literally dropped. Seeing yourself through someone else's eyes after such radical changes is something special. I was smiling from ear to ear, feeling immense joy at how far I had come. Then, when we started talking, I told him my whole story. He reminded me that he had told me before how important it was to watch my diet, and his words confirmed what I had come to realize: 80% of success in weight loss depends on proper nutrition, and only 20% comes from physical activity. It was a reminder that the key to success lies not just in workouts but also in how you eat. At that moment, I understood that I wasn't just on the path of physical transformation, but I was undergoing a deep restructuring of my lifestyle and mindset.

Practical advice: Physical exercise without the right diet may be less effective. If you truly want lasting results, be sure to focus on what and how you eat. Proper nutrition is the foundation for successful weight loss and maintaining fitness.

From that moment on, I approached my diet and exercise with even greater awareness. Every day, it got easier, and I continued to lose weight and improve my physical shape. But what was most surprising was how my food preferences changed. I used to love fried and fatty foods, but now those foods no longer brought me any pleasure. In fact, they made me feel uncomfortable. After 2-3 months of healthy eating, my taste buds completely reset, and I began to enjoy simple, natural flavors. It was like a rebirth: foods that used to seem boring or bland now brought me real joy. My body was cleansing itself, not only physically but also in how it perceived food — it was an amazing discovery that made healthy eating not an obligation but a source of pleasure. Every healthy meal filled me with a sense of lightness and harmony, and I began to see food as an ally on my path to health.

Practical advice: When transitioning to healthy eating, give yourself time to adapt. At first, it may seem like food is less flavorful, but over time your

taste buds will reset, and you'll start enjoying simpler, healthier foods. This will help you stay motivated and stick to your new lifestyle without feeling deprived.

Following my trainer's recommendation, I started doing water aerobics, and it became my true salvation. The water had an incredible effect on my body. Water aerobics was gentle on my joints and muscles while still allowing me to work out effectively, toning my skin and keeping my muscles in shape. This was especially important for me because I was still prohibited from heavy physical activity due to my surgery. Water aerobics was an excellent replacement for intense workouts, and I felt my body becoming stronger and more toned with each session. In addition to this, I began to regularly undergo massage courses — every six months, I had 10-12 sessions. Massage helped improve circulation, restored my skin, and relaxed my muscles after workouts. This comprehensive approach allowed me to achieve results that I couldn't have reached with regular workouts alone. The feeling of lightness and strength that the water gave me became a new stage of recovery, a source of joy and confidence in my abilities.

Practical advice: If you need gentle physical activity, water aerobics is an excellent option. It helps strengthen muscles, improve skin condition, and keep the body toned without straining your joints or spine. It's the perfect choice for those recovering from surgery or with health restrictions.

In the summer of 2023, I moved to another city, and this

became another important milestone in my life. Moving to a new place always brings changes, and in my case, it affected not only my daily routine but also my physical activity. I decided not to delay getting back to workouts and signed up for a local gym. In the new city, I met a new trainer, and this became a fresh experience for me. He introduced new training approaches that were different from what I had tried before. This new approach gave me extra motivation because every workout revealed something new. I started noticing how my body was changing: the flat butt I had after losing weight began to take on more rounded shapes, and my skin was becoming more elastic. My physical abilities expanded, and this gave me confidence. I began to feel that my body was coming back to life and regaining its strength. By this time, my weight had stabilized at 123 pounds, and I started focusing on improving muscle tone and endurance.

Practical advice: If you have the opportunity to try something new in your workouts, don't be afraid to experiment. A new trainer or different program can provide a fresh perspective on your workouts and inspire new achievements. Regular changes in your routine help prevent monotony and keep you motivated.

However, as important as the workouts were, they didn't always come easily. If before I had to focus on losing weight, now the emphasis shifted to building muscle mass. This turned out to be a difficult task, especially because my body hadn't yet fully recovered its strength after the significant weight loss. Increasing the weight of the training equipment, constantly pushing my limits, and occasionally feeling tired — all of this became a challenge for me. But I kept working on myself. My main motivation was knowing that despite the difficulties, I could achieve my goals if I continued to push forward. With every new exercise, I convinced myself that a strong will and determination would help me overcome any obstacles. Despite fatigue and physical difficulties, I found the strength to keep going because I knew the results would be worth it, and my body would only get better. Those moments when you feel like you're at your limit, and then push past it, brought me a sense of triumph that is hard to put into words.

Practical advice: Building muscle mass and maintaining physical fitness takes time and patience. Don't expect quick results, but stay motivated and persistent. Even small improvements over time can lead to significant changes. The key is not to give up when things get tough.

Over the years since my hospital stays, I lost an additional 37 pounds, stabilizing my weight between 119-123 pounds. This wasn't just a result; it was my personal triumph over all the challenges I faced. My body had endured all these transformations, and I was incredibly grateful for that. Over time, I accumulated a wealth of knowledge about nutrition, exercise, and my body, which I had tested in practice. Now I can intuitively control what and how I consume and understand how it affects my health and physical shape. This isn't just about rules or a diet — it has become a philosophy of life, where every decision I make is conscious and aimed at maintaining health, balance, and harmony with myself. I realized that my goal is not just to maintain physical fitness but to find joy in the process of taking care of myself. The path I've traveled has become a source of strength, and now I see each day as an opportunity to further strengthen and improve my life.

Practical advice: Listen to your body and learn to respond to its signals. Over time, you will begin to understand what works best for you. Regular exercise and proper nutrition can become not just an obligation but a source of joy when you start feeling better, stronger, and more confident.

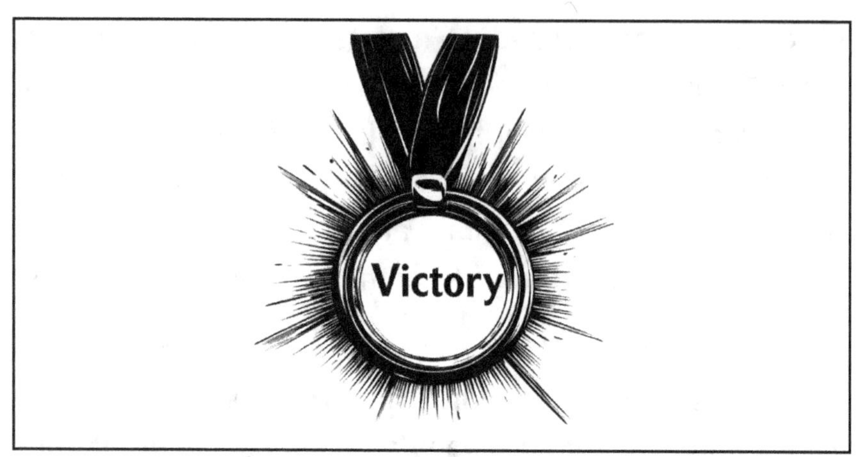

Conclusion — «Well, here we are at the end (spoiler: I won, how about you?)»

And here I stand, at what seems to be the end of this journey. But you know what I've realized? There is no real end. This journey, full of struggles, discoveries, disappointments, and unexpected victories, will always continue. The path to knowing yourself is not a destination; it's a lifelong process. When I look at my reflection, I don't just see a slimmer woman. I see someone who went through her own personal hell, someone who at one point stood on the edge between wanting to give up and the determination to take control of her life. I see a woman who has learned to respect her body and soul, who, through the struggle, has found harmony within herself. And although my journey was full of obstacles and pain, each challenge became a stepping stone upwards, strengthening my resolve and belief in myself.

When I reflect on my past, I don't feel regret. I don't regret what happened, because every fall, every mistake taught me something important. These were lessons, albeit tough ones, but they helped me understand the value of self-care. However, I also understand that many of the problems I face today could have been prevented. If I had started taking care of myself sooner, I could have avoided many of the issues I now deal with on a daily basis. Chronic pancreatitis, which requires constant monitoring, physical changes that I feel in my body — all of this is the result of years of ignoring my body's signals, years of putting myself second instead of making my health a priority.

But what if I had started sooner? This question haunted me for months. Could I have avoided these consequences? Maybe. But you know what's most important? You have the chance to start earlier. You have the opportunity to do what I couldn't — prevent, instead of fix. Don't wait for your body to start sending out warning signals. Start acting now. Every action you take today is a promise that your future will be brighter and healthier. This journey, no matter how hard it seems, is the future you are creating with your choices today.

When I think about how my life has changed, I don't just see the lost pounds. Losing 123 pounds is just a number, but behind it lies emotions, experiences, fears, and most importantly, transformation. The weight is gone, but along with it went the fears, doubts, insecurities, and bad habits.

I'm no longer the person I used to be. My transformation took years — in the first year, I lost 55 pounds, and then over the next two and a half years, I shed the remaining 68 pounds. It was a slow but inevitable process of change that affected not just my body, but my mind. I changed, step by step, realizing that each pound wasn't just a number on the scale, but a symbol that I was moving forward.

Each of those pounds is a symbol that I took a step toward a better life. But it's not really about the numbers. What's most important is how I feel today. This isn't just a victory over excess weight. It's a victory over myself, over my own limitations, fears, and insecurities. And I want every one of you to understand: you can achieve the same. You're capable of more than you think. Even when it feels like everything is falling apart, you have a strength inside you that you might not even be aware of yet.

When I look back on my journey, I see every small victory, every moment when I wanted to give up, but kept going. And that is the foundation of my success. I've realized that we are capable of much more than we can imagine. Even when it seems like everything is collapsing, there is strength within us that we haven't yet unlocked. I found this strength in myself when I thought I couldn't go any further. And it gave me a confidence I'd never had before. A confidence that even in the toughest moments, I can find a way to keep moving forward.

The second important lesson I've learned is that we and

our bodies are one. We too often try to fight our bodies, ignore their signals and needs, forgetting that our bodies are always trying to help us. Our body is our main ally, not our enemy. I've learned to listen to my body, to understand its signals, and to take care of it. And that has changed everything. Instead of fighting, I've learned to work with my body as a team. Now, my body and I move in the same direction. We're no longer opponents in this game, but partners striving for a common goal — health and harmony.

Change doesn't happen quickly, and I've learned that any transformation takes time and effort. We live in a world where everyone wants instant results, but the truth is that real change happens slowly. It might seem hard and frustrating, but that's exactly what makes the process of change real. Every small step is an investment in a better future. And each of you can take that step today. You don't have to wait for a miracle. You need to become that miracle for yourself.

And finally, the most important thing I've learned on this journey is that your life is your responsibility. No one can do it for you. No one can force you to change until you want to do it yourself. Taking care of yourself isn't selfish; it's essential. And the sooner you start, the more you can do for yourself. Don't put your life on hold. Don't wait until it's too late. Make caring for yourself your priority right now. You only have one life, and it belongs to you.

This book isn't just a story about how I lost weight. It's the story of how I found myself. And I want you to understand: this journey is possible for everyone. I started late, but your journey can begin right now. Let it be filled with joy, discovery, and self-love. The main thing is to take the first step and not be afraid of change. Every day is a new opportunity to be better than you were yesterday.

Remember: you are your biggest priority. When you're in harmony with yourself, everything around you starts to change. And that is the real victory. When you start to value yourself and your health, you'll notice how your surroundings, your goals, and your life begin to transform.

Now, standing here, I can confidently say: I won. It was a long road, but it was worth it. And each of you is capable of the same. The key is not being afraid to take the first step. Victory isn't a destination, it's a process. And if you decide to take that journey, you've already won. Victory is every day when you choose to care for yourself, when you put your health and well-being first.

Don't stop at what you've achieved, always set new goals. And don't get stuck on just one task — look at the bigger picture and act, considering all the factors. Having reached my target weight, I understand that this is only the beginning of my journey, my new path, and the new me. I've become not just a slim girl again (though, judging by my age, you could call me a woman), but I've gained a stronger character and a clearer understanding of what I want from this life. Realizing that I was able to overcome something as big as obesity without magic pills, spells, or surgeries is truly empowering and gives me strength for new accomplishments and life plans.

During these years, even before I reached my target weight, I met my current husband. I love him, and he loves and supports me in all my endeavors. I've made new friends and acquaintances who were initially surprised at how I didn't eat from the common table, but then they stopped paying attention to it. Although, to be honest, some still try to feed me. But they do try to make something from the dishes I eat.

And part of these people, after learning my story, were the ones who encouraged me to write this book to give motivation and support to others who are still on their journey to a new version of themselves.